STOP INSOMNIA!

STOP INSOMNIA!

HOW TO SLEEP WELL
THROUGH BED EXERCISES

RICHARD R. FULLER

Illustrated

Exposition Press   *Smithtown, New York*

FIRST EDITION

© 1980 by Richard R. Fuller

ISBN 0-682-49582-4

Printed in the United States of America

To the first pupils of the Sleepwell System,
whose enthusiasm has encouraged me
to write this book

Contents

Introduction

This book was written for the one million people who take sleeping pills every night and for the two million more who suffer from insomnia, but are fearful of habit-forming tablets. Doctors are undecided as to whether it's worse to lie in bed tossing and turning, or to obtain artificial oblivion with sleeping pills.

The problem exists because the phenomenon of sleep has not yet been fully explained. Despite massive research, for example, it's not understood why people feel wretched without slumber and on top of the world after a good eight-hour sleep.

One important theory suggests that during our evolutionary period of development, the condition of sleep was more natural than that of wakefulness. Scientists agree that the young of many species exhibit characteristics of their forebears from ages past. For example, if you awaken a baby, it starts crying. This response may be a throwback indicating that our prehistoric ancestors preferred sleep to physical activity.

Of course, many creatures exhibit this tendency today, including mammals, reptiles, fish, and insects. In a sense, therefore, there seems to be a subconscious desire to be asleep, not awake. Once the basic needs of food and bodily activity are satisfied, it's natural to seek insensibility, and, as we shall see, some aspects of this concept are helpful to the system of bed exercises I prescribe in this book.

Bed Exercises

We do know that a proper night's rest is the best natural medicine. Colds, headaches, indigestion, shocks—all yield to its unique healing power.

Having myself been an insomniac, I took my last bottle full of tablets and discarded it many years ago, determined to try and finish forever the necessity for drug-induced sleep. At the time, it felt to me like jumping in the deep end of a pool without being able to swim, and the first weeks I would wake up hollow-eyed and listless because of sleepless nights. Two things kept me going: an afternoon nap in the armchair and a system of elementary sleep-inducing exercises I had practiced in bed, which sometimes gave me a flicker of sleep toward dawn. The basic premise was that if one could somehow discover the most comfortable positions and remain therein with a relaxed mind and body, it would provide the most favorable circumstances for sleep.

Curiously enough, about ten years after I began my research, Nottingham County Council public health officials, quite independent of myself, put on an exhibition using dummies in beds, showing some of the many correct sleeping positions. It was praiseworthy as far as it went, but, naturally, it only touched the surface of insomnia. It presented positions but gave no exercises. Yet, it did show that someone was working on the problem.

My experiments over a number of years had only minor success. It was not until I systematically went through every conceivable position possible in which to place the body in bed, that I made some very exciting discoveries.

First, I found that some positions discouraged sleep, more were neutral, while others actually encouraged it. But assuming a single position was not enough. Sleep only occurred when a series of good postures was carried out with the utmost concentration, going from one to the other at regular intervals.

The Different Positions

Of course, this was only the beginning of the system that was to evolve, since there were numerous variations for positioning the arms, legs, body, and head. In effect, it was similar to being in a maze, with innumerable sequences and movements from which to choose. Yet, once you learned how to get order out of chaos, you went quickly through the system, to find healthful sleep at the end.

So, the wonderful prospect came to me of being able to fall asleep speedily at will, like those two giants of history, Napoleon and Churchill. One could fall asleep while in the saddle, the other during lulls in critical cabinet meetings. When refreshed, both men dealt effectively with mighty problems of war and peace.

Why were these two able to fall asleep at will without any instruction or special knowledge? Undoubtedly, it was because of their supreme powers of intense concentration on a single subject at any given time, whether it was a campaign, a treaty, or desire for a sound sleep. Genius always finds a way!

Most people, however, find concentrating on this scale altogether impossible. Speaking for myself, it was only when I employed this new combination of controlled movements and thoughts—known as the "Sleepwell System of Bed Exercises"—that I, too, found myself falling asleep at will, night or day, like these great men.

How to Begin

You may question if it is possible for a normal person badly suffering from insomnia, but otherwise alert, to go to bed, start doing these exercises, and fall asleep while actually in the middle of them. My considered reply is yes; my experience with insomniacs shows virtually no failures.

I remember well my own first big success with the exercises. I had been to a yuletide season late evening dinner, which was an insomniac's horror of a meal and the hardest test of all to face. Peaceful sleep seemed impossible following platefuls of roast turkey, ham, sausages, Christmas pudding and minced pie, cheese, nuts, and a cup of black coffee. I resigned myself to an uncomfortable night of indigestion and nightmares because of my indiscretion.

But the next morning, it was only when I awoke

after doing the exercises, and leaped out of bed with a happy burst of song, that I jerked to an astounded stop when I suddenly remembered all the heavy food I had consumed. My first real attack on sleeplessness, with the aid of the exercises, worked—I'd had eight hours' glorious rest on an overly full stomach. Even more important, all my fears about insomnia vanished henceforth. I can assure you, this gives one the greatest feeling of freedom in the world.

Obviously, it would not be wise to eat on such a scale every night, but by following a sensible diet daily, one is able to enjoy the celebrations that come to us all.

That event took place years ago, and since then I have done a few minutes of bed exercises while comfortably tucked under the blankets each night, and I can honestly say they have never let me down.

In effect, I decide what I eat, drink, and enjoy in life without apprehension of what's going to happen after dark. Naturally, the benefit of these nonmedical exercises to my general health has also been one hundred percent for the good. Those day-to-day maladies that we all catch never have the opportunity to grow into anything serious following successive nights of sound sleep. Most ordinary illnesses yield to the system's supreme healing power.

All Forms of Insomnia

Over the years the Sleepwell System has overcome many forms of insomnia, especially helping sleepers in the coldest conditions of winter, or those kept awake by worries and foreboding that plague the

xiv   INTRODUCTION

mind and become magnified in the long hours of darkness.

In addition, like many other people, I was particularly unable to sleep in hotels and during long journeys, whether by train, plane, or car. Naturally, this spoiled holidays in the past, but through the use of the advanced exercises specifically designed to deal with the above difficulties and detailed in this book, I can literally sleep my way through anything.

Yet while readers' techniques become equally as good as they progress, they must remember the basic principles remain the same. A bed exercise is simply a move and a hold, however complicated it later appears.

Your Program

How do the following chapters instruct one in learning a system that has taken twenty years to evolve, and how long will the process take?

The course is divided into four sections. Take one section a month, doing the bed exercises in the appropriate chapter of the book, while peacefully reposing under the covers, and beginning as soon as you switch off the light. Sleep usually comes quite quickly, and if you should awaken during the night, redo the exercises.

At the end of the first month, proceed to the second section, gradually getting better at the techniques, then proceeding to the third and fourth sections. The complete system takes four months, at the end of which time (providing you have reasonably followed the instructions) you will be an accomplished sleeper, able to slumber tranquilly under both normal and adverse conditions.

After the four sections have been completed, dispense with doing bed exercises every night, for you should be able to sleep well without them, retaining them only for emergencies.

In addition to the above benefits, the book offers instruction on how to overcome that greatest of all hindrances to rest—the ghastly noise menace of modern civilization.

No book about sleeping would be complete without helpful information for those who can't sleep together properly. During the old-fashioned double-bed days, couples invariably reposed in harmony; there was far less sleeplessness in the land. But new times require new methods. By doing bed exercises together in the special manner explained in chapter six, this happy state can be recaptured.

I firmly believe that after completing the four-month course successfully, former insomniacs will not only throw away their sleeping pills, but their general health will markedly improve because of the abundance of sound slumber.

In conclusion, the book further explores the exciting realm of sleep by showing that as it is possible for one to control sleep, so can one control dreams. Chapter seven will help readers comprehend the close link between sleeping when they like and dreaming what they wish, a technique that involves superimposing a series of dream-control exercises on the bed exercises.

STOP INSOMNIA!

1

Section One: Laying Your Foundation for Sleep

The bed exercises for the first month are the easiest of the course, but they are also the most important.

Once you acquire sufficient skill at making the elementary bed movements correctly, you will be ready for the advanced exercises of the following sections. The foundation of good sleep depends on this four weeks of practice.

Keep at them nightly until the exercises become smooth and free flowing. Apart from being of little use, awkward, jerky movements can result in covers falling on the floor, which is not conducive to sound

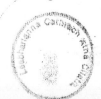

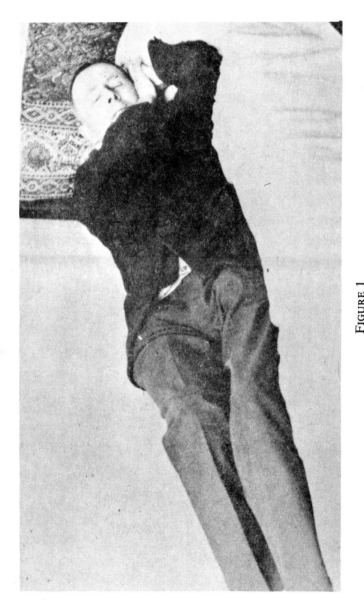

FIGURE 1

The wrong way—a night in this position, and you're on the road to the land of depressed insomniacs.

sleep. Get your basic changes and position right, and the complete system will follow naturally.

How to Begin the Exercises

The bed exercises consist of a series of combined physical and mental exercises done to varying sequences and patterns. The technique is to get into the correct position and hold it for a certain length of time, then move on to the next position. Each move and hold is a bed exercise.

Begin as soon as you get into bed, and redo the exercises if you should awaken during the night. (I rarely find it necessary to start again now, as I seldom wake up once asleep.)

In effect, you "attack" the problem positively. Just passively waiting for slumber has never helped anyone. By following the system prescribed, you forget about weary tossing and turning because you are too busy concentrating on your exercises.

Good postures induce sleep; bad ones discourage it (see figure 1). Usually, one good position is not sufficient; but, if a series of positions is used in the correct sequence, healthy sleep comes involuntarily and normally with little waiting.

Exercise One

Exercise one is quite simple and one of the most important in the system (see figure 2). After twenty years, I still do it as soon as I get into bed.

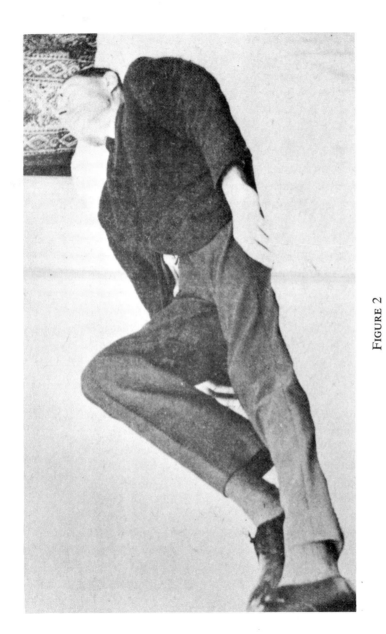

FIGURE 2

The right way—Mr. Fuller maintains that ten minutes in this position, and you're well on the way to the Land of Nod.

simple, but together not as easy. It usually takes a month's practice to gain proper control.

You have now been in bed for twenty minutes. There's no need to look at the time—you have computed it mentally. Having gone this far, you may feel you would like to move or turn over. You must avoid movement at all cost. Instead, finish the exercise, which consists of a double repeat, i.e., another two hundred breaths, in and out, in the same position, for a total of fifteen minutes.

Practice makes perfect, and you should do it accurately, but you may find you're making mistakes. Either your enumeration may be wrong, or you may forget your breathing routine. You're indulging in long, sleeplike sighs. Of course, you don't realize it, but sleep is gripping at both body and mind.

By the time the month is finished, you will not reach two hundred often.

The Degree System of Movement

Figure 3 shows the eight main positions of sleep in degrees. Basically, all the tossing and turning and other contortions of bad sleepers can be reduced to these positions. In exercise one you started at the 90° position, looking up at the ceiling. After fifteen minutes you turned in a circular counterclockwise movement to the 0° position.

The positions of 45°, 135°, 180°, and 270° are used as you progress. All exercises are done between the 0° and 270° positions, both clockwise and counterclockwise. At these points reverse and come back. By not using the sector between 0° and

270°, you keep the covers in order and avoid disturbance.

Of course, one doesn't travel around the positions like clockwork. Normally, when making a turn, you move into the position that appears most comfortable and likely to bring sleep. This varies throughout the night.

Performing the "Star"

The "star" is a variation in the bed exercises. It's a technique for focusing concentration during an exercise. It consists of missing a number and doubling back on it, usually done in the middle of the exercises.

As you approach 50, e.g., . . . 45, 46, 47, 48, jump to 50 and then back to 49 and then on to 51. The sequence is . . . 45, 46, 47, 48, 50, 49, 51, 52. . . .

Execute a "star" only in the middle of the exercise and, of course, remember your breathing throughout. It gives a twinkle or "star" effect along your pattern of enumerating. It corresponds to the start or jump you often get when you are falling asleep.

Exercise Four: The Turn

Make a full movement from 0° to 180° in one sweep and finish facing the opposite wall. The internal organs of the body are differently poised in relation to one another, and you'll feel greatly relaxed, and sleep should be very near.

Continue practicing the above exercises for the full month. You will then be ready for the more advanced exercises in chapter two.

Keep a Diary of Sleep Habits

Progress will be improved by keeping a record of each night's events during the four months of the course. You can then pinpoint errors, analyze why some nights are bad and others good, and record periods of sleeplessness, indigestion, outside noise, worry, and so on. (*See* the "Diary of Sleep Habits" on page 12.)

Copy the headings on four sheets of paper, one for each month of the course, leaving enough space to fill in the results for each night. Enter your answers first thing in the morning while they are still fresh in your mind.

Finally, maintain a daily graph of the Total Hours Sleep column. Should it not keep at a steady level, check back on the points in the above paragraphs and take the appropriate remedy in conjunction with the advice in chapter five.

DIARY OF SLEEP HABITS

Monday (date)

Time of last meal[a]:	7:00 P.M.
(light-1; medium-2; heavy-3)	2
Digestive trouble (nil-1; slight-2; acute-3)	1
Noise or disturbance (nil-1; slight-2; acute-3) (explain)	2
Time turned out the light	10:30 P.M.
Time started exercise one	10:31 P.M.
Time techniques bring sleep	11:00 P.M.
Sleepless periods (if any) in order of occurrence[b]:	
First	1
Second	0
Third	0

Tuesday (date)

Time of final awakening[c]:	7:00 A.M.
Time of rising	7:30 A.M.
Total hours in bed	9
Total hours of sleep	7
Events of previous day (average-1; above average-2; exciting-3)	2
Events of coming day (average-1; above average-2; exciting-3)	1
Feeling on arising (fresh-1; above average-2; dull-3)	1
Remarks	Good-quality rest

Note: All times taken from exercises only. Do not consult watch or clock.

[a]Exclude bedtime drink.
[b]Calculate by working back.
[c]Over fifteen minutes but not over thirty, mark 1. Over thirty minutes but not over sixty, mark 2. Over sixty, mark 3.

2

Section Two: Planning a Complete Night's Rest

You are going to progress still further in mastering insomnia in this section. In an ideal world, and sleeping under perfect conditions, things would be less difficult, but we frequently have to sleep through times of ill health, worry, distress, or uncomfortable surroundings, especially when away from home. It is then that good rest is a real boon, hence the need for more advanced presleep exercises that "stick" and are not forgotten.

Note: Continue the following to section four; then return to simple exercises.

The exercises thus far, having served their purpose of providing sound sleep, are no longer necessary to do every night. The enumerating, positioning, and breathing techniques of the system are put in reserve, and one reverts to normal sleeping habits again. A few selected guidelines are all that's needed to sleep well in the future. Meanwhile, practice the exercises in strict rotation, and take an extra month if required for proficiency.

These Techniques Induce Planned Sleep

Having thoroughly practiced the special breathing and enumerating methods in section one, you are ready to go ahead with the following exercises.

Of course, if you are able to sleep well most nights without any further exercises, do not start them. Keep them in mind for the sleepless nights that come to us all.

Exercise Five

If you do the following fifteen-minute exercise without error, you will sleep through almost anything. In my case, I allow up to three errors; should I make more, I then realize I am not attacking sleep; when less, I am rarely awake to finish it. Although lying almost still throughout the duration, it is something of an art to complete successfully.

Return to the 180° position described in exercise four. Turn counterclockwise until you are in the 0° position. Pause a moment to check for steady breathing and prepare to count to a hundred. The exercise enumeration is not sequential as before, but split up, consisting of forward, reverse, miss, and pick up, and so on, in time with your breathing. It is a technique to induce planned sleep.

First, divide the 100 into three subsections of 30 each, leaving 10, and enumerate your subexercises as follows:

1 to 10 . . . straight, then 11, 12, 13 . . . followed by 20, 19, 18 . . . (reverse).

Next, 21, 22, 23, 24, 25 . . . pick up 14, 15, 16, 17 . . . and finish 26, 27, 28, 29, 30.

Continue without pausing or moving into the second subexercise, which is different:

30 to 40 . . . straight, then 41, 42, 43 . . . followed by 50, 49, 48 . . . (reverse).

Next, 44, 45, 46, 47 . . . and finish 51 to 60 . . . straight.

The third subexercise is a repeat of the first:

61 to 70 . . . straight, then 71, 72, 73 . . . followed by 80, 79, 78 . . . (reverse).

Finally, 81, 82, 83, 84, 85 . . . pick up 74, 75, 76, 77 . . . and finish 86, 87, 88, 89, 90.

To deal with the 10 over, go straight through 91 to 100.

Commit this to memory to get the rhythm and then do it smoothly with few errors. Two aids are: keep your mind projected slightly ahead of the counting in readiness for the variations as they occur, and avoid having to catch your breath as you go over the complicated parts. Think forward!

It is vital always to carry out the techniques to the best of your ability. The brain is most susceptible to sleep at the beginning of an exercise, so try particularly hard as you begin each one. Even if sleep does not immediately result, you are laying the foundation for success in the next one.

Surprising as it may seem, trying to be on the alert for voluntary mistakes does not keep people awake very long, and the involuntary ones mean sleep is forthcoming. Just waiting helplessly is of little use.

Choosing More Good Positions

There is a choice of three different positions at 0° or 180°. You may choose lying straight, slightly bent, or curled up into a ball. Finding the right position helps sleep considerably, and my advice is to start in a bent posture that you hold for the duration of the exercise. Later in the night, try others by selecting the one which seems most comfortable at the time.

In the 90° position there's still a choice, despite the necessity of resting on the back with a straight trunk. One or both knees may be bent and, if desired, your hands may be folded across your chest.

Exercise Six

The early exercises will certainly succeed, however bad we feel, if attacked strongly, but the difficulty is that an overly full or disturbed stomach can wake us up repeatedly. Exercise six overcomes both indigestion and the excitement of late-night parties.

The remedy is to soothe and exercise at the same

time at the 270° mark. It often happens that we suffer the full onslaught of party and stomach troubles in the middle of the night. If so, finish the exercise you are doing and then do exercise six.

Positioning yourself for this exercise with ease and economy of movement requires a certain knack. Face 180° and then bring your left knee forward until It Is resting on the bed, move your left hand to the side of the pillow, and press down with your palm to lift your head. At the same time, slide your right shoulder backward and slowly down.

Finish by lying flat out with gentle pressure on your abdomen, which quickly eases a queasy stomach and makes restful sleep possible. To allow you to breathe comfortably, make sure your right arm is tucked under your shoulders with your head turned left.

It helps to press back the side of the pillow until your face rests at the edge. I keep this position during exercise three or five, and, invariably, refreshing sleep follows until morning. For those not used to sleeping on their stomach, hold the position for fifteen minutes to correct troublesome symptoms, and then swing directly back to 0°

One always strives for overkill with insomnia, and I have enough exercises to last many nights. Some, however, I have not needed for years.

Nighttime Noises Turn Many Healthy People into Insomniacs

Apartment living, neighbors' television sets, and late-night traffic are typical examples of disturbing noises. However, exercise four should overcome all but the worst disturbances. American scientists are experimenting with recordings of neutral noise which, it is claimed, drowns out raucous sound and does not interfere with sleep; it's known as "white noise." However, I do just as well simply by turning on my stereo and carrying on with the exercises.

When outside sounds become excessive, apply the practical advice found in the helpful hints in chapter five.

Afternoon Naps Are Good for You

There is always more to be discovered in a beneficial health science, and presleep exercises prove no exception.

Adapt bed exercises to daytime armchair sleep. They work as well while reclining, instead of lying horizontally. Use the 45°, 90°, and 135° positions, together with the half-straight and curled-up postures.

3

Section Three:
Sleep as You Like;
Wake-up Exercises

Now that you are acquiring the skill of being able to sleep more easily, there are many thrilling prospects ahead. Sleep increasingly becomes a servant to harness its unique power to your demands. In addition to the prevention of poor physical health, a sound sleep can halt psychological troubles by means of mood-control exercises, leading later to the actual control of one's own dreams. These achievements do not evaporate in the morning; they should be carried forward, with benefit, throughout the day.

But you must learn more advanced bed exercises

to become the master or mistress of your bed. In the previous section, readers were shown how to keep their breathing even and regular; yet, sometimes, especially when traveling and subjected to vehicular movements, it pays to do bed exercises with irregular breathing. Deliberately cause your breaths to become quick or slow and short or long to conform with new patterns of exercises.

Exercise Seven: Imitating Waves

Here is the powerful wave technique resembling the rollers beating on the seashore, first small, then big, and then small again. Together, they have a tranquilizing effect on body and mind.

Start with small waves.

1, 2, 3, 4, 5, 6, 7 . . . small and medium waves building up and breaking.

10, 9, 8 . . . (reverse) the waves slowly moving back to the sea.

11 to 23 . . . large waves breaking.

30, 29, 28, 27, 26, 25, 24 . . . the waves going back to the sea.

Repeat the pattern three times up to 100, plus ten over straight 91 to 100.

To obtain full value from this exercise relax as much as possible, and get your breathing into harmony with the waves and move with them. Gradually strengthen the depth of your breathing at each count up to the point of the waves breaking. Then when the wave has broken and is receding, reverse and breathe slowly and lightly so you come up and down in unison with the waves. It helps if you rock the body slightly in time with your breathing.

Exercise Eight: The Staccato Exercise

This exercise is the opposite of the waves, being an assault on sleep when conditions are difficult. The sequence is sharp and repetitive, and you must endeavor to keep your body rigid:

1, 2, 3, 3 . . . (staccato)
6, 5, 4, 4 . . . (reverse)
7, 8, 9, 10, 10 . . . (staccato)
14, 13, 12, 11, 11 . . . (reverse) and then straight 15 to 30 with a "star" at 25.

To deal with the 6 over, go straight on through 91 to 96. Repeat the pattern three times. You need all your willpower, and even expressing it by clenching your fists will not unduly delay the onset of sleep.

Exercise Nine: Advanced Techniques

So far our exercises have been recorded by number and are the basic techniques of the Sleepwell System. Now we add depth by using first alphabetical letters, followed by words which form pictures—all within the framework of enumeration.

Exercise nine is based on exercise three, with the addition of letters. It makes readers employ four dimensions simultaneously—breathing, enumerating, positioning, and lettering, as follows:

1 to 30, A . . . (straight)
31 to 60, B . . . (straight)
61 to 96, D . . . (straight)
1 to 30, H . . . (numbers straight, letters reverse)
31 to 60, G . . . (numbers straight, letters reverse)
61 to 90, F (numbers straight, letters reverse)
91 to 96, E . . . (numbers straight, letters reverse)
1 to 30, I . . . (straight)
31 to 60, J . . . (straight)
61 to 90, K . . . (straight)
91 to 96, L . . . (straight)

Practice exercise nine until you are as good with letters as you are with numbers. Then you are quite ready to take the big step forward in the system, which is to clothe the exercises in pleasantly evocative words and phrases. When you are half-asleep, suggestions can readily be absorbed by your subconscious mind. Precontrolled thoughts and the imagination can surface in slumber; then you not only sleep well but have happy dreams, too. This really is sleeping as you like.

Exercise Ten: Mood Control

What are the best emotive words to use to influence our thinking? They must, of necessity, be short, and the simple ones are favored, such as, *warm, well, sleepy, now, happy, holidays, pastimes,* and so on.

Everyone has different preferences, so be flexible and choose your own; the principle remains the same. Begin with numbers, then the words, as shown in this exercise:

1 to 40 . . . (straight)
Then . . . S, L, E, E, P, Y, N, O, W, G, O, L, F, T, O, M, O, R, R, O, W (repeat each letter spelled out separately, as in exercise nine)
62 to 100 . . . (straight)

Repeat the sequence twice, making it a fifteen-minute exercise, and briefly pause for cheerful memories and hopes, while spelling out each word. Remember, the enumeration provides a definite beginning and end; without this aid we would ramble on and get nowhere.

Note: Letters of one syllable are uttered on exhaling, the exception, W, being slurred as described in chapter one.

Minimum Covers with Maximum Warmth

The Sleepwell System works at its best in a cold room without heat. Scott slept soundly during polar blizzards, while the most remote and healthiest Eskimo tribes still prefer the igloo. I no longer light the bedroom fireplace, and I discarded my hot-water bottle and electric blanket years ago and have slept soundly ever since.

None of us can sleep properly when cold, but the human body generates sufficient heat to slumber peacefully during bitterly cold nights. Working on the same idea as insulation, we must trap the warm air inside the bed. The remedy is to sleep with your head under the covers, and exercise one shows this method of starting cold nights in comfort. In effect, you make the bed into a tent by pulling the covers over your head and tucking them in behind the neck; your raised right leg acts as the pole.

After fifteen or thirty minues, depending on the length of the exercise, when turning to 0°, your knee comes down. Form another tent by sliding your left arm forward, taking a piece of the sheet, and holding it against the top of your head. Then push back with your right shoulder, pulling the sheet taut, thereby erecting another snug covering. It's also a comfortable sleep position with ample space for breathing and warmth.

I use a sheet and three blankets, the bed being made so that the first sheet and adjoining blanket completely cover my head, while the top two only come up to my shoulders.

Many doctors frown upon the habit of inhaling too much raw night air. In fact, I now live significantly free of colds, and leg cramps are an agonizing pain of the past. This beneficial style of sleep does take a little practice, but, eventually, you will not be comfortable any other way. By doing the few exercises in the month allowed for this section, you will be well prepared for the worst winter nights ahead.

Wake-up Exercises

All good things come to an end, including a good night's rest. Half the world cannot get up, and the morning rush of many would be laughable, if the results were not often almost tragic. Often-heard comments like "Poor timekeeper," "Unpleasant to work with until coffee break," and "My husband's impossible in the mornings," are invariably due to the way sleep draws to a close in the early hours.

There are three problems the Sleepwell System has to overcome: waking-up, not falling asleep again, and actually getting out of bed.

No system can rouse you at exactly seven o'clock. If this is essential, you must use an alarm clock. Otherwise, the following exercises will have you up smiling on time for breakfast.

Nature signals the night's drawing to a close by dropping the body temperature in the morning to its lowest in twenty-four hours, which is enough to start us stirring for more warmth. In the summer, early sunrise and birdcalls also provide a welcome stimulus to the senses.

Do not begin bed exercises again; open your eyes wide. Remember, good positions encourage sleep; bad ones discourage it. Therefore, assume awkward positions, known as waking-up exercises. Two of my best are as follows:

Turn to 0°; lift up your body, bend your left arm behind your back, and come down heavily, at the same time twisting your neck toward the ceiling. Hold fifteen minutes.

To be certain you do not become sleepy, make a clockwise swing round from 0° to 315° into the unused sleeping sector. Finish by lying on your chest, cramped and uncomfortable, with half the covers off.

Getting up should be quite easy at any time now, and you should end the night as it was begun—in exercise one's position, lying on your back with your arms parallel to your body. Hold the position and then enumerate from 1 to 20. Promptly at 20, rise on the elbows and pause while collecting your thoughts. Then spring out of bed, ready for the day's work after a good night's sleep.

Finally, whatever your musical ability, singing a few bars of a favorite song as you arise is the greatest tonic for yourself and the household. Never get up silent.

Wake-up Tips

To avoid arousing yourself too early with wake-up exercises, always consider the following before starting:

1. Take a brief glance out the window to see whether it's getting light, according to the season.

2. Are you becoming chilly?

3. If you are still warm and darkness reigns outside, go back to sleep.

Those studying the system are requested to follow every stage with the utmost care, because the system offers a pattern of exercises that will last a lifetime and is a passport to perfect health.

4

Section Four:
Slumbering to
Your Own Sequence

During the last three months, you have progressed from the most elementary exercises to the most difficult, now possessing a large range with which you can build up your own pattern of exercises. Of course, you will not need to do the advanced exercises every night. The best way to bring sleep quickly is to construct a series of exercises to suit your own capability, according to whether you are a high-strung or placid person.

For example, you could well start with a few simple exercises, followed by more difficult ones, and then return to moderate ones. If still awake, turn the whole pattern inside out by doing a difficult one. It depends on whether you are among those who fall asleep quickly and then wake up during the night, or take a long time dozing off but then sleep till dawn. The system aims to iron out both these irregularities.

Below are important factors to consider when making up your own combination of exercises and variations:

1. What length of sequence can you personally manage without mistakes? One and a half hours, two hours, or even two and a half hours? (The longer the better when practicing the course.)

2. In the winter, position your body for warmth as described in chapter three. Consider when and where to insert the necessary movements in your sequence. The same holds true for coolness in the summer.

3. How to overcome noise problems.

4. Where to introduce exercise six on those nights it's necessary for stomach comfort.

5. Numbers, letters, words: obtaining the right mixture, including "stars" in your sequence.

6. Precautions to take with wake-up exercises, to avoid arousing yourself in the early hours.

7. A drink? A read? Stopping the sequence on a really poor night and taking a "rest period."

8. Correct timing in straight, bent, and curled-up body positions. Also fingers, hands, and elbows.

9. Getting out of bed to go to the lavatory: yes or no?

10. Avoid nose-blowing and throat-clearing, ignore pins and needles and the urge to move. Over-

come nighttime worries about business, family, health, and life in general.

The above ten points are considered and incorporated in the set of specimen exercises that follows.

Important Note

It is essential to utilize the elasticity of an exercise to the fullest because it will help bring easy sleep.

As stated in chapter one, each move and hold is a bed exercise. The next move starts a new exercise. It can be a complete turn, a half-turn, or any motion of the body, however small, while facing the same direction. But it must be decided from the start.

For example, moving your arm or leg constitutes the beginning of another exercise, and it must be held for five, ten, or fifteen minutes as planned.

Making an impromptu movement in the middle of an exercise because of discomfort or forgetfuless is a mistake and must be avoided. It is an obvious deterrent to slumber. (See chapter five for hints on avoiding mistakes.)

Exercises should be kept in sequences of five minutes, normally not exceeding fifteen minutes. Sometimes, when I am aware that sleep is forthcoming, I use a half-exercise of only two and a half minutes to do the trick. Occasionally, when extra self-discipline is required, I use an exercise of thirty minutes without movement. Make your own exercises short, medium, or long to suit your own needs.

The Model Sequence for Insomniacs

The model sequence takes one hour and forty-five minutes from the time I turn out the light until the time I finish the last exercise. If required, the timetable can be extended another half an hour without discomfort. Normally, I don't get nearly that far and am asleep within fifteen minutes.

Time passes rapidly even when doing the longest sequence. There's none of the dreary eternity of a bad night, and a half an hour of exercise seems like five minutes.

The pattern starts as follows: exercise one (fifteen minutes); exercise two; and exercise three (thirty minutes, i.e., enumeration of three hundred, then repeated).

At the end of this period I am lying on my left side, facing the wall, and have been in bed a total of forty-five minutes (see section one).

As far as position, I decide on the intermediate half-bent body position for this exercise: right hand lightly closed, left-hand fingers straight and resting on the bed.

A quarter of the way through exercise three, I insert a "star" to avoid daydreaming, thus focusing my attention on the counting, e.g., 45, 46, 47, 48, 50, 49, 51, 52 . . .

Again, when three-quarters through, I perform a "double star," e.g., 45, 46, 47, 48, 51, 49, 50, 52, 53 . . .

I'm not asleep yet, but the outlook is hopeful, as I now find myself yawning and making involuntary mistakes because I'm almost dropping off.

The moment arrives for exercise four, and after making the turn and facing the opposite wall, I get ready for an all-out attack on sleep through exercise five.

My position is curled up, with both hands lightly clenched. I get as far as . . . pick up 74, 75, 76, 77 . . . ,

when the neighbor's door slams, and I'm wide awake
again.

Undaunted, I repeat exercise five and again become drowsy; the time comes for the next move, which
is the turn back to 0°.

Tonight I decide it's necessary to employ section-
three techniques, utilizing letters and emotive words.
Therefore, I omit exercise seven and do exercise nine
for a count of three hundred and then go straight
on to exercise ten, using the word and sentence method
as described, position as before. Readers, of course,
should have already chosen their own suitable phrases;
the principles are the same.

This is the outline of the sequence and its ter-
mination, in the rare event of being awake. I have
been in bed one hour and forty-five minutes. Having
rested quite still and controlled during this period, I
am feeling remarkably composed.

Should I feel sleep is imminent, I can make
another turn and then repeat exercises nine and ten
for an extra half-hour. If still awake, I would stop the
exercises temporarily, taking a rest break and other
remedial measures as described in chapter five.

5

Helpful Hints

When and How to Relax during the Exercises

Many insomniacs find relaxing most difficult, especially at night, when vainly awaiting sleep. Total relaxation for the one and a half hours of a complete sequence is impossible and is itself no guarantee of slumber. But letting the limbs go limp during five minutes in a single exercise is quite simple, even for tense people, and provides a big boost toward sleep.

For instance, in the model sequence starting with exercise three, it's wise to do the first five minutes normally and not try to relax. Then unwind fully in the second five minutes, returning to normal in the third.

To relax properly, first loosen your shoulders, then your arms, and so on down your body to your legs and toes. Let yourself go weak all over if possible. Particular parts to check are around your eyes, your jaws (unclench your teeth), the pit of your stomach, and your hands. Breathe slightly slower than normal.

Relax like this once or twice in each half-hour. I find such looseness very helpful in the last five minutes of a sequence, for the reward at the end usually is sound sleep. Of course, avoid making mistakes in your enumerating while relaxing.

Becoming Taut Helps, Too

In contrast to relaxation, immobility is an equally important element of the system. Five minutes' time with your body stiffly poised provides a sharp counterpoint to relaxation, and this is when the highly-strung individual can catch up with the more placid readers.

The tense person can "attack" the problem of insomnia wholeheartedly in this particular phase; by now we know that just passively waiting never gets results.

Thus, at the appropriate moment, tighten the body into almost rocklike immobility. Stop everything that moves; your breathing should be sharp and deliberate. Some parts of the face are nearly always moving, so attend especially to your lips, tongue, eyes, and nostrils, to be sure they are still. Also, cease all mouth, throat, and digestive sounds to the greatest possible extent. It's like an exaggerated form of exercise one, and it can easily be done for five minutes.

Actually, when feeling a little below par in my general health (and we all get this way at times), I do this wonderful exercise for half an hour, and again if I awaken during the night, and feel all the fresher the following morning.

Clearly, clenching your fists and tightening your jaws, and so on would never bring sleep. Yet when done for very brief spells before relaxing, the reaction from one to the other hastens success toward the end of a sequence.

Stretch Normally

Stretching is the most common form of rest, and it includes breathing naturally. Assisted occasionally by relaxation and tautness, it's all that's required for a good night's sleep.

Every exercise, of necessity, is carried out in one of the above three states. To select the right one, use the following muscular signals:

Normal: Lightly depress thumb of right hand. This indicates it's to be an ordinary exercise.

Relaxed: Depress first finger of right hand.

Immobile: Depress second finger of right hand.

Hold the body in one of these ways to prevent aimless drifting. Apply the signaling device at the count of twenty-five. The reason for this is you are too occupied at the start of an exercise, and you minimize the chance of error by deciding later.

Try Slower Breathing

Resist the tendency to breathe quickly in your effort to fall asleep. It's due to anxiety, and is neither good for the heart nor conducive to sleep.

The three-second rule for one complete breath is the custom, but when on the brink of sleep, the insertion of a really slow rate in the sequence brings success.

Every exercise in the system may be done in this fashion. For instance, using exercise three, at normal speed one hundred breaths take five minutes. Adjust to a slower rate, so that seventy-five take the same amount of time.

Of course, arriving at seventy-five in the enumerating, you jump the gap to one hundred . . . 71, 72, 73, 74, 75 . . . 100 . . . and begin a new exercise.

When breathing in this manner, allow the exhalations to be long and tranquil, ending with a sigh and pause. Remember, it was more natural to our earliest ancestors to be dormant than active.

When next sharing a bedroom or dormitory with others, listen to the many different breathing styles of people asleep. It's simple to pick out the particularly restful sleepers and imitate their slow breathing.

Avoid Too Many Mistakes

With all my years of sleep experience, I still make errors in the sequences. I am not referring to the involuntary ones no one can avoid when oblivion is close, but the careless ones caused by inattention to details and daydreaming.

There was a time when I believed the exercises were to blame for a bout of sleepless nights. It was only when I checked and found as many as six errors in a single exercise, that I realized the system itself was not wrong. I discovered that when I stopped making mistakes, normal sleep returned.

So, it is important to concentrate on the exercise; otherwise sleep will be retarded. Common mistakes are enumerating incorrectly, failing to hold positions, and inaccurate signaling. Whether the errors are physical or mental, both are equally damaging. Therefore, the earnest would-be sleeper must keep a tight grip on the situation until the subconscious takes over.

But we must be realistic; even the best of us can't always be a hundred percent accurate. The problem is solved by allowing up to three mistakes per turn. If less, so much the better. Tests show that this permissible figure does not affect the early onset of sleep, but, if exceeded, you probably won't sleep well.

Referring to the model sequence, it contains three turns, meaning there's a total of nine allowed before proper rest is interfered with.

To find out and correct what may be causing the trouble, signal your errors using your left hand, i.e., move your thumb for mental errors, and the index finger for physical errors.

Controlling Your Eyes, Nose, Mouth and Diaphragm

Eyes. Remember not to open your eyes during or between exercises. Rest your gaze downward; this is the normal angle of vision.

The eyelids should be gently closed to avoid "fluttering," because this is the equivalent of the hopeless "tossing and turning" of the muscles in the optic region. During the night, these tiny movements assume huge proportions and divert your full attention from the exercises.

The cure is simple. Now you know about it; watch yourself while carrying out the exercises. This healthy relaxation of the eyes causes one to feel all the fresher the next morning.

Nose. Nasal obstructions and colds present obstacles to correct breathing and steady enumerating.

The remedy is to take a large handkerchief, folding it several times and placing it between your mouth, your nose, and the pillow. Keep your mouth open temporarily and carry on with the exercises. In this way, the pillow remains unsoiled, and the extra effort needed to do the exercises properly does only good. The excellent sleep that follows means an end to the cold, too!

Mouth. Avoid tightness in your mouth. At the beginning of each exercise, be sure that your jaws are not rigid, your lips are only lightly pressed together (except with a cold, as above), and that the top and bottom teeth remain slightly apart. Your tongue should be touching your lower teeth lightly. Check that the above points are correct simultaneously and maintain throughout.

At the count of a hundred, pause to briefly clear your throat and swallow if necessary. Normally, this habit disappears in time as you complete the system.

Diaphragm. Using the diaphragm consciously and properly not only benefits sleep, but also your general physical health. This large muscle at the base of the lungs lowers and raises with each breath, forcing air in, then out and, obviously, should be utilized to the fullest extent.

It's excellent for controlling slumber, since your breathing immediately becomes steady. Too few people deliberately use their diaphragms in this manner. By lying flat on the bed and breathing and expelling deeply, you have visual proof of your breathing by observing the chest expanding and the stomach contracting.

Therefore, from now on inhale as instructed, especially when you begin your nightly exercises. The golden rule is to breathe through your nose with the conscious assistance of the diaphragm.

Rest Periods

During the first twenty-five counts of each exercise, focus thoughts on eyes, nose, mouth, and diaphragm. After that forget them, for control should soon become automatic. In any event, you have the exercises themselves to attend to.

You have realized by now that there are many exercises and aids in the system to bring sleep. Each alone has a useful though limited effect, but the cumulative results of a large number eventually cause the insomniac to break through the barriers to slumber.

Understandably, however, we must make provision for the worst case of insomnia. After completing a sequence without sleep, it's advisable to have a rest. The system is not designed as an endurance test which, clearly enough, would not bring sleep. I personally rarely need a break, but it's available if necessary for the sleepless night even some skilled sleepers occasionally suffer. It's all the easier to get to sleep after stopping the exercises for thirty minutes and then starting again.

During the rest period, I suggest you make yourself comfortable for a while. Sit up in bed, sip a drink, or read a few pages of something light to take your mind off the exercises. As soon as your rest period is over, lie back refreshed and ready to tackle the next sequence.

The rest period also is very useful for combating excessive outside noises such as a neighbor's party or television. Frequently, these noises stop or lessen before the half-hour is over. If not, start a fresh sequence, especially utilizing exercises seven to ten, and rigorously avoid mistakes. If performed correctly, you'll forget what's going on outside. The judicious use of earplugs or cotton appreciably assists by muffling outside disturbances.

Getting up to Use the Lavatory

I would not advise leaving bed for this purpose too often. Years ago, when I was an insomniac, I used to get up at the slightest urge, and the habit seriously interfered with my sleep. There was the rest lost the half-hour before, and also the time getting drowsy again afterward. Once you give way like this, you are in and out of bed at least once every night.

Therefore, resolutely refrain from getting up for this purpose and concentrate on the exercises. At first, the urge will not completely vanish but remain in the background. After completing the system, you will find you have overcome this disability.

The same principle applies to nose-blowing. With many people, it's a nervous habit that can be similarly overcome, with remarkable improvement in your sleeping performance.

Naturally, if you are in any doubt about your health, you should first check with your doctor before cutting down on late-night visits to the lavatory. The same advice applies to all other exercises for the course.

Sleeping without the System

Now we come to the stage where readers will reap the maximum benefit of the system, because they can begin sleeping at will, without using the exercises.

I find it difficult to believe that for years I had worked conscientiously at them when it was no longer really necessary.

One night I made the astonishing discovery that I could sleep well without any concentration. It felt something like having bandages removed from a healed wound, except I had no doctors and nurses to tell me when to do so. As the pioneer of the system, I had to find it out the long way around!

Naturally, as with any kind of recovery, one cannot just forget the problem; one has to take a few sensible precautions to see it does not reoccur. This is done by employing a rudimentary sequence which will keep you on course so that you continue to sleep extremely well, as well as insure you retain the knowledge of the full system in reserve for a rainy day.

Basically, what happens is that instead of exercises

and sequences, a series of blanks is substituted. The sleeper continues with the same system but relies on abbreviation and instinct, something he is now well qualified to do. Enumerations, "stars," letters, emotive words, and like techniques are dispensed with for the most part.

For instance, referring to exercise three in the model sequence in the previous chapter, it consists of a count of one hundred; to change it into a blank exercise, the enumeration becomes as follows:

1, 2, 3, 4, 5 . . . 95, 96, 97, 98, 99, 100

From 6 to 94 stop enumerating, but breathe normally:

. . . 1, 2, 1, 2, 1, 2 . . . (1 on inhaling and 2 on exhaling)

At 95 pick up numbering again, having approximated the five minutes as accurately as possible, and finish off the exercise to 100.

It takes about the same time as the real exercise of five minutes, and experienced people get within a few seconds' accuracy, which is all that's needed.

Continue with the second exercise in similar fashion:

101, 102, 103, 104, 105 . . . 195, 196, 197, 198, 199, 200, stopping, counting, and picking up as before.

In this manner, the sequence is turned into a dummy with the mental effort reduced to minimal proportions. The practitioner is left with the outline of the sequence.

However, transforming the lessons and maintaining them as an effective instrument of sleep is a little more complicated than forming blanks. The prime target, despite the new simplicity, remains sound sleep.

We have to retain the main principles, or there's a danger of reverting to aimless tossing and turning and becoming an insomniac again.

Accordingly, there are "built-in" safeguards to the blank system, including many of the physical positions and movements continued below.

Having successfully completed section four, readers should now make the changeover to the blank system.

New Blank System Derived from the Original Model

Turn back to chapter four and check the step-by-step differences as they occur.

First, determine the duration of the sequence. Personally, I find one hour and fifteen minutes quite sufficient, instead of the previous hour and forty-five minutes.

The pattern starts as before:

Exercise one (fifteen minutes—unchanged)

Exercise two (unchanged)

Exercise three (fifteen minutes—carried out in blank form)

1, 2, 3, 4, 5 . . . 95, 96, 97, 98, 99, 100, leaving out the enumerating and picking up as described.

Repeat twice, making for a total of fifteen minutes.

Now relax your limbs and move for comfort, but remain in the 0° position, facing the wall. This brief motion permits you to start a fresh fifteen-minute exercise which is part blank and part original model as follows:

For the first ten minutes continue with two blanks as above, then finish off with five minutes of original exercise three, including full enumerating, making a big effort to break through the sleep barrier as you come up to the finish . . . 95, 96, 97, 98, 99, 100.

If awake, carry out exercise four and continue with a new dummy utilizing exercise three again for thirty minutes in the manner detailed. Once more, include five minutes of the full model, and this time insert a "star" for concentration.

On those nights when sleep is really elusive, complete the sequence by returning to 180° and finish off with a fifteen-minute blank.

Useful Tips

1. Mistakes happen easily in the blank system. Try not to exceed three per turn, as before.
2. Apply the relaxing, taut, and normal techniques together with the signaling time at twenty-five. In this case, approximate it.
3. After a month, the rhythmic . . . 1, 2, 1, 2, 1, 2, 1, 2, 1, 2 . . . tends to become blurred. So take care to do it a minimum of five times per exercise, slowly and consciously. If you forget, count it as one mistake.
4. Carry out the complete original model once every six months to keep in practice.
5. Now you should be sleeping involuntarily without even needing the blank system. When this happens, fill in any brief waking gaps with dummies.

"Ticking over" Peacefully

On weekends and holidays we often lie in bed late. Sleep's finished, but it's too early for breakfast.

Try not to spoil a good night's sleep by tossing and turning before getting up. "Tick over" by remaining still, closing your eyes, and breathing normally;

... A, B, A, B, A, B ... (without enumerating)

If you should fall asleep again, so much the better. This rest method is, of course, not an exercise. It can also be applied to keep oneself fresh during long train or car rides.

6

How to Sleep with Your Partner and Enjoy It

The insomniac's partner never knows whether he or she is coming or going at night. If one sleeps well and the other tosses and turns, one of them is bound to get irritated. If they toss and turn together, the bed creaks, the covers come off, and, after a short spell, neither really wants to get into a double bed again.

Of course, if both are insomniacs, the two toss and turn until it's time to get up. Either way it's a mixup, and we all get a hearty laugh at the pair when portrayed on television or in movies. Unfortunately, to real-life couples it's a problem that causes much marital unhappiness. Now the knowledge gained by bed exercises will enable them to sleep together properly.

Start This Way

The best thing to do is establish a set of exercises that will avoid troubling one's bedfellow. Then one of them sleeps as usual, and the other by means of bed exercises; everything is peaceful. Let's adapt the original model sequence to this purpose.

First, the insomniac, say the husband, must decide on which side of the bed his wife should sleep. With our particular pattern, he must get in on the left side with his wife on the right. The objective is, with the assistance of an early exercise, to turn away from his wife into his own corner, meaning less disturbance to both, and carry on from there.

Exercise one (fifteen minutes—unchanged). In this position one cannot interfere with the other. Of course, before switching off the light, the partners must be reminded about the eyes-closed, no-speaking rule.

Exercise two (unchanged). Since exercise one is approximate, it's gentlemanly to synchronize your first turn through 90° with one of your wife's uncontrolled movements, thus minimizing interference.

Exercise three (thirty minutes—unchanged; but see section on points of contact below).

Now, retire into your shell for the night, forget everything but the system, and carry out the sequence as if you were alone. Carefully proceed through the various postures, correct breathing, enumerating techniques, "stars," degree movements, and the like to exercise ten.

Points of Contact

A few attitudes must be modified according to circumstances, as the following examples show:

You can't curl up into a ball or stretch out, unless your wife's got her back to you or happens to be doing the same. Hence, it's wise to stick to the half-bent positions as much as possible.

The warming-up techniques can't be employed because they would entail taking much more than your share of the covers. However, two bodies together produce more than enough warmth for any winter's night, so the omission of this exercise does not make any significant difference.

The digestive turn is easily practiced when needed, as it means swinging right away on to the edge on your side. However, I recommend you use it only after festive eating events and not daily.

The long-term remedy is to have well-regulated evening meals that don't interfere with rest. In this connection, apply the tips on healthful eating habits at the end of the chapter.

The wake-up exercises still serve admirably if your wife usually gets up first to make breakfast. Start these exercises after she's left the bed. Of course, on the mornings when you arise first, this would not be right as it involves having most of the covers on the floor. If this is the case, use an alarm clock.

Although doing the system requires keeping

strictly to yourself, because it's sleep you want, eminent sociologists maintain that body contacts and caresses do contribute to marital happiness; deep human instinct causes one to touch one's partner. The trouble is, arms and legs are heavy, while fingers, toes, hot breath, and hair are distracting when carrying out exercises. What can be done?

When facing each other, keep your distance, but if you're behind come close and rest your left arm on your thigh (not hers), and then bend the right arm up and lightly place your hand against her shoulder. It's a reassuring contact, and you can easily keep it there for the duration of an exercise. Similar light touches can doubtless be tried by readers.

Whatever the degree of one's insomnia, it's advisable to employ the full model system instead of blanks, when first starting these curative measures with a partner alongside. You certainly need all the concentration aids available. After you have acquired skill in the new situation, revert to the dummy exercises as before.

People who sleep in double beds must now ask themselves the question: Shall we both cooperate when doing the exercises?

If the answer is yes, so much the better, and I suggest the two of you begin exercise one in unison and harmony. The better sleeper has no need to do the enumerating parts; just loosely follow the physical movements and stay clear of your partner. As the insomniac turns to 180°, the other also moves in the same direction. This synchronizing of the movements makes it all agreeable and provides a fine beginning.

But suppose one partner, say the wife, will not

help and decides to make a nuisance of herself in bed. Clearly, at first, bed exercises will not teach the husband how to withstand a sudden knee in the buttocks in the middle of the night, or a whipping away of the sheet and blankets in the cold bedroom air.

However, nature is so strong that when necessity really arises, one can sleep through practically anything, like lying in a water-logged ditch or standing up in a freezing, drafty corridor. Stranded travelers and prisoners of war vouch for this astonishing fact.

Therefore, ignore interruptions from whatever direction, because before long you will be sufficiently versed to sleep through anything. If your partner switches on "Home on the Range" or "Alexander's Ragtime Band," then you sink deeper into the realm of sleep. The main thing to look forward to is that eventually the most difficult partner succumbs to the natural appeal of sleep through bed exercises, and you will enjoy doing the system together.

Tips on Healthful Eating

1. The all-important stomach—forget you have such a thing, especially at nightfall.

2. Never overeat or undereat.

3. Have your main meal at midday.

4. Eat a light dinner or supper, and complete any remaining eating and drinking necessary by eight o'clock. This allows you to go to bed with a calm body.

5. Always masticate food slowly, and finish one mouthful at a time. Sit upright, and don't cross your legs at the table. These rules may appear elementary,

but a glance in a crowded restaurant shows how few follow these excellent precepts.

6. Finally, remember that a sound digestion depends on using a small amount of willpower over what sort of food we eat. There lies the road to good health as well as good sleep. Therefore, follow a reasonable diet that agrees with you. If in doubt about certain food values, consult your doctor or visit your public library for information on the subject.

7

Dream Control
through Bed Exercises

I was having one of those pleasant dreams about an old friend; then it vanished when I suddenly woke up. Having departed in real life, she did so again in my dreams.

That incident occurred many years ago, before I began using the system, yet now I can bring her back, as well as other past happenings in my life, for the most part whenever I like. The ability to plan in advance, through bed exercises, can actually allow us to have those "pleasant dreams" we wish our loved ones at bedtime.

It is natural for you to wonder if you, too, can choose a subject or person close to you, tuck yourself

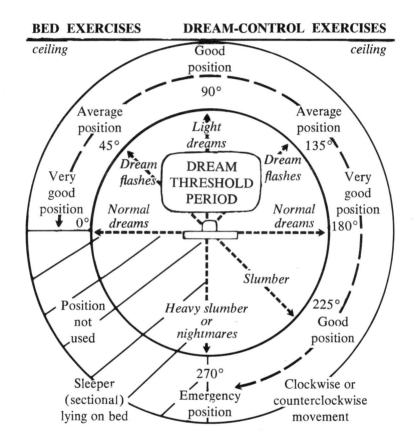

FIGURE 4
The dream threshold

in, and then await with confidence all your dreams
come true in the brilliant kaleidoscope of slumber.

It can be accomplished, and readers with us from
the beginning of this book appreciate the close link
between sleeping and dreaming as we like. However,
before beginning this specialized method, it's wise to
consider all the implications.

It's said that a little knowledge can be a dangerous
thing, and dream control should not be practiced by
people who only want to experience cheap thrills or
to dwell on nostalgic memories. At first, I blundered
in wanting all my dreams to contain exciting images
of riches, totally opposite from my normal way of
living. Before long, this Jekyll-and-Hyde sleep had a
bad effect on my health. I awoke unrefreshed and un-
willing to face the usual events that confront us daily.

My advice, therefore, is to avoid harmful themes,
and stress the wholesome things in life; dwell on the
holidays, your health, your work, your freedom, on
faith, on hope, on happy memories, and on your
family. There's good in each of us; unfortunately, it
is often submerged our entire lifetime. With sustained
practice, controlled dreams can draw out this quality
and bring it forward into our daily existence with
inestimable benefit.

How to Enter the Dream Threshold

The outer circle of figure 4 show the bed-exercise
positions with which we are already familiar; the
inner circle shows those that control dreams. It's
simple to see at a glance the relationship that exists
between the two. For example, 90° is both a good

sleeping and light-dreaming position. The technique involves switching from bed exercises to dream-control exercises at the proper moment. This transfer takes place during the threshold period as indicated, which only lasts a fraction of time. It's then you're taught how to plant the seeds of your desired dream in your mind, as you fall asleep.

Dickens was a great believer in the powers of sleep and dreams to influence us for good or bad. In *Oliver Twist* he wrote, "It is an undoubted fact that although our senses of touch and sight be for the time dead, yet our sleeping thoughts, and the visionary scenes that pass before us will be influenced—and materially influenced—by the mere silent presence of some external object."

In order to be in control from the start, there are a number of preparations which must be made, including the requirements mentioned above, before and after going to bed. If not carried out with extreme care, nothing will happen, or, when you do fall asleep, you will only half-dream. We all know this unsatisfactory state, and it's as far as you will get if you do not prepare carefully. Of course, this poor state of sleep does not possess any of the therapeutic health value offered by true dream control.

Exercises in Dream Control

I like to exercise dream control about once a month to keep in practice, and I use the help it gives me to make life generally more agreeable.

First, I decide the type and intensity of my chosen dream for that particular night. A good night's dream to me (someone who feels the cold during winter) bathes me in the tropical sun and warm seas of the Canary Islands, where I have spent some glorious holidays. Before going to bed, I put on an extra blanket so that my dormant mind will become more attuned to thoughts of these sunshiny islands.

I always begin the night at the 90° mark, using exercise one for a full fifteen minutes. But this time, I don't want to risk falling asleep on my back, because, as the pointer shows, I would only have light dreams, and I want them to be more intense. Accordingly, on this evening, I start with a shorter bed exercise of five minutes at 90° to become slightly drowsy, before turning counterclockwise to 0° for the double onslaught on sleep and dreams.

One more simple bed exercise, employing exercise three for fifteen minutes, brings me closer to slumber with a calm mind. Readers now enter the crucial phase during which the changeover occurs from one system to the other. This is the time when conscious thoughts recede, and the subconscious mind starts to come forward. At one hundred enumeration, this threshold period is imminent, and the moment quickly arrives when neither mind is in control, and the brain is left briefly in limbo, which I define as the place where forgotten things collect.

It is then ready to receive and assimilate the autosuggestion we have prepared. Being able to judge the right instant means mastering the art of successful control. If performed too soon, we wake up with a start, something we all have experienced. If performed too late, sleep certainly comes, but it's either disappointingly dreamless, or about another subject altogether.

The average threshold period lasts fifty counts—two and a half minutes—and only then do dream-control exercises work well. Obviously, it requires considerable willpower, as well as experience, to be able to imprint, when barely awake, the image of the dream directly on the exposed subconscious by spelling the letters for my particular objective:

. . . C, A, N, A, R, I, E, S . . . into the enumeration and breathing—C during the first inhalation, A the second, until the end.

The sequence takes 8 × 3 seconds—twenty-four seconds—and I repeat it while my mind is in the threshold period, at the same time conjuring up happy memories.

There should be just enough time to cross-spell the suggestive keyword "warmth" as follows:

. . . C, W, A, A, N, R, A, M, R, T, I, H, E, S . . . and as the seconds finish, the subconscious takes over completely, and the vision of the chosen dream arrives on the scene.

Readers only get a wonderful opportunity like this once a night, and they will not succeed except in their first sleep. It's unwise even to make another attempt the same night, as it imparts an anxiety neurosis that interferes with rest.

Other favorite dreams of mine are about simple home blessings and absent loved ones. In the latter instance, it is helpful to have and hold an article of clothing, like a glove or a keepsake.

Surprisingly, there is little need to consider color, for dreams appear before us like pictures in black, white, and gray. The Encyclopaedia Britannica tells us that only in very rare cases do sleepers report having dreamed in color. It would seem that some of the more vivid sensory nerves do not operate during sleep.

Of course, with two sharing the bed, and one or both desiring to dream of the other, you cannot do better for an external aid than follow nature, and utilize light hand contact, as described in the previous chapter, prior to the threshold period, Then spell and cross-spell your names and other endearments, during that period.

As the diagram indicates, the intensity and length of dreams for the most part are controlled by position. For quick flashes the choices are 45° and 135°; slumber is best promoted at 225°.

The 270° mark, as we know, is fine for sleep during a digestive emergency, but it's unwise to apply dream control at the same time. The chosen subject would likely produce a nightmare.

Practical Aids toward Control

Much depends on regular hours and sensible meals; late dinners should be avoided. Readers who are now conforming to the diet tips in chapter six should not be troubled by nighttime indigestion.

Precisely recording your dreams is a more elusive task than attaining the skills in sections one to four. One cannot expect immediate results as with the latter, obviously because it takes longer than bed exercises to master the more difficult techniques. When you start practicing, it's a good plan to keep a dream diary like the one for recording sleep exercises. Write down, under various headings, brief descriptions of length, intensity, details, connection with previous day's events, and so on, either at night or first thing in the morning, before such details are forgotten. Then study your progress over the first few months.

You will often discover, on referring to your diary, that a particular dream was based on an incident that happened in your life some weeks earlier. Examples of mine include the rare sight these days of a horse in the streets, and dreams about racing, a clergyman and the church, a train and a visit to London. It's the aim of dream-control exercises to reduce the time lag to a single night.

If initial progress seems slow, maybe you will do better if you began exercises at the 45° or 135° positions for quick flashes, and proceed to longer dreams from there. Choose a favorite but simple subject in the beginning, and work up to more elaborate ones as you progress.

No exercises yet devised can do more than start you off at scene one of your chosen dream. Those following depend on fantasy, health, and your own personality. Results come according to how well sleepers make the changeover from one exercise system to the other. It's perseverance that narrows the waiting gap.

Whatever the early outcome, the exercises do insure plenty of sound sleep, and there's little doubt that readers who do them regularly will eventually succeed with dream control, too.

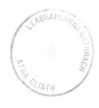